TYPE 2 DIABETES BOOK

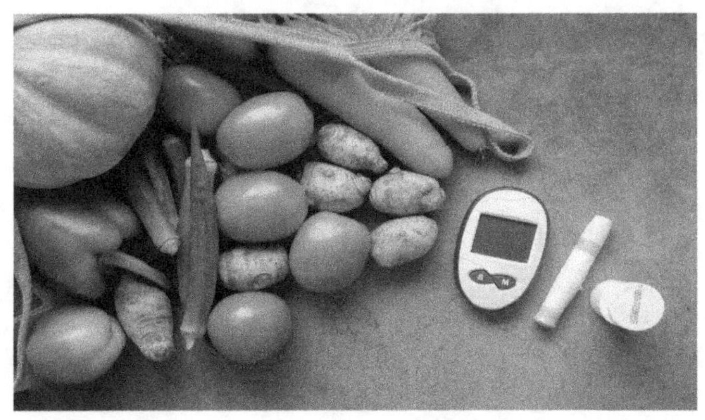

The Sage's Approach to Understanding and Reversing Insulin Resistance.

Crystal Kyle

TABLE OF CONTENTS

INTRODUCTION

In the quiet neighborhood of Maple Grove, lived a woman named Sarah. She was a cheerful soul, always ready with a smile for her neighbors and a warm meal for her family. Little did she know, a silent intruder was creeping into her life – Type 2 diabetes.

It all started with a seemingly innocent cupcake. Sarah, with her love for baking, often indulged in creating sweet delights for her family and friends. One day, after savoring the joy of her latest creation, she noticed an unquenchable thirst that no amount of water could satisfy. Puzzled, she dismissed it as a temporary quirk, perhaps the aftermath of a particularly delicious treat.

As weeks passed, an unwelcome companion joined the unrelenting thirst – fatigue. Sarah, once brimming with energy, found herself grappling with a tiredness that seemed to settle into her bones. It wasn't the weariness that comes after a busy day, but an exhaustion that lingered like a stubborn dog, clouding the vibrancy of her daily life.

Soon, the bathroom scale became an unexpected adversary. Weight loss, a mystery disguised as a blessing, accompanied Sarah's journey. Friends noticed the change, expressing concern, but Sarah, caught in the whirlwind of denial, shrugged it off as

the result of a newfound fitness routine. Little did
she realize that her body was sending distress
signals that could no longer be ignored.

Then came the pain – an unexpected and
bewildering sensation in her feet. It started as a
tingling, a subtle discomfort that soon escalated
into a constant, throbbing ache. Each step became
a reminder of an invisible force tormenting her, a
pain that seemed to have taken residence in her
very foundation.

A routine checkup unraveled the mystery. Sarah
was face to face with Type 2 diabetes. The doctor's
words hung in the air, heavy with a reality that
Sarah hadn't anticipated. "You have diabetes," he
said, and suddenly, her world shifted.

The diagnosis was not just a medical revelation; it
was a seismic shift in Sarah's life. Diabetes, an
uninvited guest, now demanded a seat at every
table, a voice in every decision. The pain she felt
was not just physical; it was a deeply emotional
struggle. Sarah grappled with guilt, wondering if her
love for sweet indulgences had led her down this
path. The diagnosis wasn't just about managing
blood sugar levels; it was about navigating an
emotional labyrinth, where every step carried the
weight of an unforeseen challenge.
The daily routine that once felt like second nature
transformed into a series of calculations and

considerations. Sarah found herself juggling medication, dietary choices, and the constant vigilance that diabetes demanded. Yet, amidst the struggle, a different kind of pain emerged – the pain of adjusting to a new normal, of redefining what it meant to lead a healthy, fulfilling life.

As Sarah walked this uncharted path, her story unfolded as a testament to resilience. The pain she felt was a silent anthem echoing the struggles of countless individuals facing Type 2 diabetes. In the heart of Maple Grove, where stories of triumph and tribulation were etched into the fabric of everyday life, Sarah's journey became a beacon of hope.

Her pain became a catalyst for change, not just in managing the physical aspects of diabetes but in reshaping her relationship with health and well-being. It was a narrative of learning, adapting, and discovering new found strength in the face of adversity.

In the simplicity of Sarah's tale, there lies a universal truth – that Type 2 diabetes is more than a medical condition; it's a personal journey. It's a journey that encompasses not only the physical challenges of blood sugar management but also the emotional roller coaster that accompanies the diagnosis. Through the pain, Sarah found resilience, and in her story, we find a reminder that even in the face of life-altering challenges, the

human spirit has the capacity to persevere and
come out stronger on the other side.

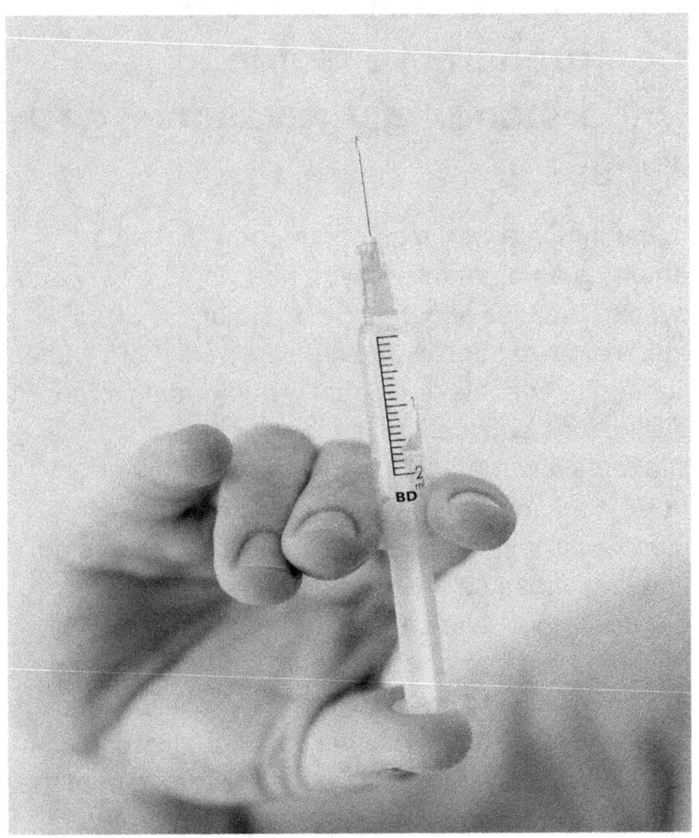

CHAPTER ONE

DECODING DIABETES -A Comprehensive Guide to Understanding, Prevalence, and Types.

In the intricate workings of our body, diabetes emerges as a notable player, affecting the way our system handles sugar, known as glucose. This guide aims to simplify the concept of diabetes, shed light on its prevalence globally, and untangle the distinctions between its primary types.
Diabetes is a metabolic condition where the body faces challenges in regulating blood sugar, or glucose. Imagine your body as an intricate system where glucose serves as essential fuel for cells. In diabetes, this balance is disrupted. In Type 1 diabetes, the immune system mistakenly attacks insulin-producing cells, resulting in insufficient insulin. Type 2 diabetes involves a dual struggle – cells resist insulin, and the pancreas can't meet the increased demand. This creates elevated blood sugar levels, impacting overall health.

Understanding Diabetes: The Glucose Story

Diabetes is like a traffic jam in the body's energy highway. Picture glucose as tiny cars navigating through our bloodstream, providing fuel for the cells. Normally, insulin acts as the traffic cop, helping glucose enter the cells where it's needed. In diabetes, this traffic control system gets a bit wonky.

In Type 1 diabetes, it's as if the traffic cop (insulin) is on a break because the immune system mistakenly attacks and takes out the insulin-producing cells in the pancreas. Without enough insulin, glucose can't properly enter the cells.

Type 2 diabetes, on the other hand, involves a double challenge. Firstly, the cells become a bit stubborn and don't respond well to insulin's instructions. Secondly, the pancreas, the organ responsible for producing insulin, is working extra hard but often can't keep up with the increased demand. This creates a situation where glucose struggles to get into the cells, leading to a buildup in the bloodstream.

Prevalence of Diabetes: A Global Puzzle

The International Diabetes Federation (IDF) tells us that in 2021, around 537 million people were living with diabetes globally. That's a lot of individuals navigating their own traffic jams in the body's energy highway.

Diabetes doesn't play favorites; it's found in various corners of the world, impacting communities both big and small. The prevalence of diabetes is influenced by a mix of factors, including the way we live, our genetics, and the natural aging process.

In this era of fast-paced living, with more time spent sitting and less time moving, the risk of developing Type 2 diabetes has gone up. Urbanization, changes in eating habits, and the allure of processed foods have all played a part in the rise of diabetes. What's interesting is that this isn't just a challenge for well-off countries; it affects places with different levels of development.

Types of Diabetes: Unraveling the Varieties

Understanding diabetes involves knowing there's more than one type. Let's look at the two main ones – **Type 1 and Type 2.**

Type 1 Diabetes: The Immune System Mix-Up

In Type 1 diabetes, the immune system, usually a superhero defending against invaders, goes a bit haywire. It mistakenly targets and attacks the insulin-producing cells in the pancreas, creating a shortage or even a complete absence of insulin.

Who It Affects: Often shows up in childhood or adolescence, catching individuals early in life.

What Happens: Without sufficient insulin, glucose struggles to get into cells, leading to increased levels in the bloodstream.

Type 2 Diabetes: The Double Trouble Dance

Type 2 diabetes is like a dance where the cells aren't quite getting the moves. Cells become resistant to insulin's charm, making it harder for glucose to enter. At the same time, the pancreas is working overtime but often can't keep up, resulting in elevated blood sugar levels.

Who It Affects: Usually diagnosed in adults, but lifestyle factors are bringing it to younger individuals too.

What Happens: The cells aren't fully cooperating with insulin, and the pancreas is putting in extra effort, creating a situation where glucose has a tough time entering cells.

Why Understanding Matters

Understanding diabetes isn't just about knowing how it affects our bodies. It's about recognizing that people from all walks of life, across the globe, are dealing with this challenge. It's a call to action for communities, governments, and healthcare providers to work together in raising awareness, providing support, and finding ways to ease the traffic in our body's energy highway.

In conclusion, diabetes is like a storyline with different characters – glucose, insulin, and our body's cells – all trying to play their roles. By understanding the prevalence and types of diabetes, we gain insight into the challenges individuals face and the collective efforts needed to address this global health puzzle.

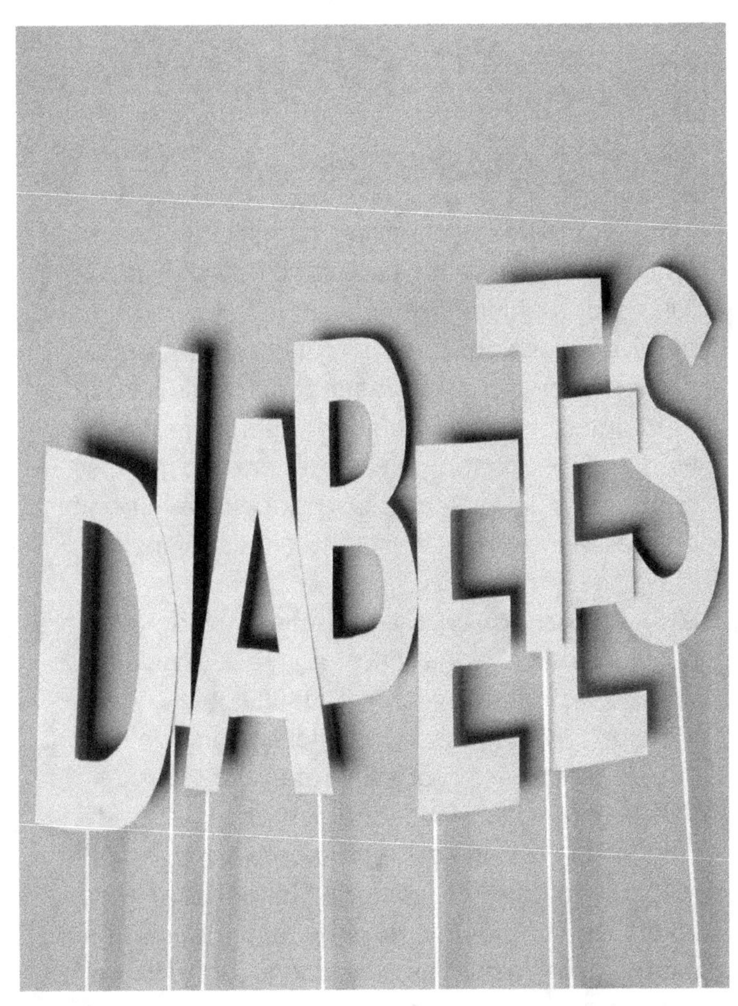

DIABEETS

CHAPTER TWO

TYPE 2 DIABETES

Type 2 diabetes is a chronic condition characterized by high levels of blood sugar (glucose) resulting from insulin resistance and relative insulin deficiency. Insulin is a hormone produced by the pancreas that helps glucose from food enter cells to be used for energy. In those with type 2 diabetes, the body either cannot produce enough insulin to keep blood glucose levels within normal ranges or it rejects the effects of insulin.

Risk factors for type 2 diabetes include obesity, physical inactivity, genetics, age, and ethnicity. While it typically develops in adults, it is increasingly diagnosed in children and adolescents, largely due to rising obesity rates.
The progression of type 2 diabetes typically starts with insulin resistance, where cells fail to respond to insulin properly, leading to higher blood sugar levels. To combat this resistance, the pancreas first makes extra insulin as a compensation.. However, over time, the pancreas may become unable to keep up with the body's increased demand for insulin, leading to insufficient insulin production. This results in elevated blood sugar levels, a hallmark of diabetes.

Symptoms of type 2 diabetes can include increased thirst, frequent urination, fatigue, blurred vision, slow wound healing, and recurrent infections. However, some people may have no noticeable symptoms, especially in the early stages.

CAUSES OF TYPE 2 DIABETES

Modernization

The rise of type 2 diabetes is intricately linked to modernization and the accompanying changes in lifestyle, diet, and environment. Several factors associated with modernization contribute to the increased prevalence of type 2 diabetes.

- **Sedentary Lifestyle:** Modernization has led to a more sedentary way of life, with technological advancements reducing the need for physical activity. Sedentary behavior contributes to obesity and insulin resistance, key risk factors for type 2 diabetes.

- **Unhealthy Diet**: The availability of processed foods high in refined carbohydrates, sugars, unhealthy fats, and low in fiber has become widespread in modern societies. These dietary patterns can lead to weight gain, insulin resistance, and ultimately, type 2 diabetes.

- **Urbanization:** Urbanization has led to changes in dietary habits, with increased consumption of calorie-dense, low-nutrient foods and a decline in physical activity. Urban environments often lack opportunities for physical exercise, making it harder for individuals to maintain a healthy lifestyle.

- **Stress:** Modern lifestyles often involve higher levels of stress due to factors such as work pressure, financial concerns, and social demands. Chronic stress can contribute to insulin resistance and the development of type 2 diabetes.

- **Environmental Factors**: Exposure to environmental pollutants, such as air pollution and endocrine-disrupting chemicals, has been linked to an increased risk of type 2 diabetes.

- **Genetic Predisposition**: While genetics plays a role in type 2 diabetes, it is the interaction between genetic predisposition and environmental factors associated with modernization that largely drives its prevalence.

Overall, the shift towards modernization has created an obesogenic environment characterized by poor dietary choices, physical inactivity, and increased stress levels, all of which contribute to the rising incidence of type 2 diabetes in contemporary societies. Addressing these factors through public health interventions and lifestyle modifications is crucial in mitigating the burden of type 2 diabetes.

Nutrition

Nutrition plays a significant role in the development and management of type 2 diabetes. Several dietary factors contribute to the onset of this condition:

- **High Sugar and Refined Carbohydrate Intake**: Diets high in sugar and refined carbohydrates, such as white bread, sugary beverages, and sweets, can lead to spikes in blood sugar levels, contributing to insulin resistance over time. Excessive consumption of these foods is associated with an increased risk of developing type 2 diabetes.

- **Low Fiber Intake:** Diets low in fiber, typically found in fruits, vegetables, whole grains, and legumes, are linked to an elevated risk of type 2 diabetes. Fiber helps regulate blood sugar levels by slowing down the absorption of glucose and improving insulin sensitivity.

- **Unhealthy Fats:** Saturated and trans fats found in processed foods, fried foods, and high-fat dairy products can contribute to insulin resistance and inflammation, increasing the risk of type 2 diabetes. Conversely, consumption of healthier fats, such as those found in nuts, seeds, avocados, and fatty fish, may help lower the risk.

- **Excess Caloric Intake**: Consuming more calories than the body needs, leading to weight gain and obesity, is a major risk factor for type 2 diabetes. Overeating, particularly of energy-dense foods with poor nutritional value, can contribute to insulin resistance and metabolic dysfunction.

- **Poor Diet Quality**: Overall dietary patterns characterized by a lack of variety, excessive intake of processed foods, and insufficient intake of nutrient-dense foods like fruits, vegetables, and lean proteins, can contribute to the onset of diabetes type 2.

- **Lack of Meal Timing and Portion Control**: Irregular meal timing and large portion sizes can disrupt blood sugar regulation and contribute to insulin resistance. Consistent meal timing and appropriate portion control are important aspects of managing blood sugar levels in individuals with or at risk of type 2 diabetes.

In summary, poor dietary choices characterized by high sugar, low fiber, unhealthy fats, excess calories, and poor overall diet quality are significant contributors to the development of type 2 diabetes. Conversely, adopting a balanced diet rich in fiber, healthy fats, and nutrient-dense foods can help prevent and manage this condition.

Low fat scare

The "**low-fat scare**" refers to the widespread dietary recommendations during the late 20th century that emphasized reducing fat intake, particularly saturated fat, as a means to improve overall health. However, this approach led to unintended consequences and may have contributed to the rise in type 2 diabetes prevalence for several reasons:

- **Increased Consumption of Refined Carbohydrates:** As people reduce their intake of fats, they often compensate by consuming more carbohydrates, particularly refined carbohydrates like white bread, pasta, and sugary snacks. These foods can lead to spikes in blood sugar levels, contributing to insulin resistance and the development of type 2 diabetes.

- **High Sugar and Low-Fat Products**: Many low-fat products on the market replace fat with sugar or other high-glycemic carbohydrates to improve taste and texture. Consuming these products, which were often marketed as "healthy," contributed to increased sugar intake and adverse effects on blood sugar regulation.

- **Impact on Insulin Sensitivity**: Low-fat diets may adversely affect insulin sensitivity. Some research suggests that diets high in healthy fats, such as those found in nuts, seeds, and avocados, can improve insulin sensitivity and blood sugar control. Thus, the demonization of all fats, including beneficial unsaturated fats, may have contributed to insulin resistance and the development of type 2 diabetes.

- **Role of Dietary Fat in Satiety:** Fat plays a crucial role in satiety, helping people feel full and satisfied after meals. By reducing fat intake, individuals may have been more prone to overeating or snacking on high-carbohydrate foods, leading to weight gain and increased risk of type 2 diabetes.

- **Disruption of Hormonal Regulation**: Dietary fat intake can influence hormonal regulation, including the secretion of insulin and glucagon, which are key players in blood sugar control. Low-fat diets may disrupt these hormonal pathways, contributing to metabolic dysfunction and insulin resistance.

In summary, the low-fat scare and the subsequent increase in consumption of refined carbohydrates and low-fat products may have played a role in the rising prevalence of type 2 diabetes. Moving forward, a balanced approach that emphasizes the quality of fats, carbohydrates, and overall diet composition is crucial for preventing and managing type 2 diabetes and promoting overall health.

CHAPTER THREE

PERSONAL ROAD TO TYPE 2 DIABETES

The personal road to type 2 diabetes is a complex journey influenced by a multitude of factors spanning genetics, lifestyle choices, environmental exposures, and socioeconomic circumstances. Understanding this path requires examining various stages and contributing factors along the way, from early life influences to the development of insulin resistance, pre-diabetes, and ultimately, overt diabetes. By exploring each stage in detail, we can gain insight into the interconnected mechanisms driving the progression towards type 2 diabetes and identify opportunities for prevention and intervention.

Genetics and Early Life Influences

The journey towards type 2 diabetes often begins with a genetic predisposition. Genetic factors can influence an individual's susceptibility to developing insulin resistance, impaired glucose metabolism, and eventual diabetes. Family history plays a crucial role, as individuals with close relatives affected by diabetes are at higher risk themselves due to shared genetic vulnerabilities.

Additionally, early life influences, including intrauterine conditions and maternal health during pregnancy, can shape future diabetes risk. The concept of fetal programming suggests that adverse intrauterine environments, such as maternal obesity, gestational diabetes, or undernutrition, can "program" the developing fetus for increased susceptibility to metabolic disorders later in life. Low birth weight, often indicative of poor fetal growth and nutritional status, has been associated with an elevated risk of insulin resistance, obesity, and type 2 diabetes in adulthood.

Lifestyle Choices and Environmental Factors

As individuals grow older, their lifestyle choices and environmental exposures play a pivotal role in shaping their risk of developing type 2 diabetes. Sedentary behavior, poor dietary habits, smoking, and excessive alcohol consumption are all modifiable risk factors that contribute to insulin resistance, weight gain, and metabolic dysfunction.

Dietary patterns characterized by high intake of processed foods, refined carbohydrates, sugars, and unhealthy fats promote inflammation, oxidative stress, and dyslipidemia, further exacerbating insulin resistance and increasing diabetes risk. These dietary habits are often influenced by socioeconomic factors, food availability, cultural norms, and marketing influences, making it challenging for individuals to adopt healthier eating patterns.

Urbanization and modernization

This has also contributed to the diabetes epidemic by promoting sedentary lifestyles, unhealthy dietary habits, and environmental exposures that increase diabetes risk. Urban environments often lack opportunities for physical activity, access to fresh and nutritious foods, and green spaces conducive to active lifestyles. Socioeconomic disparities further exacerbate these challenges, as individuals from lower-income communities may face greater barriers to adopting healthy behaviors and accessing healthcare services.

Environmental factors such as exposure to air pollution, endocrine-disrupting chemicals, and other pollutants have also been implicated in the development of insulin resistance and type 2 diabetes. Chronic exposure to environmental toxins can disrupt metabolic homeostasis, impair insulin signaling, and promote adipose tissue inflammation, contributing to **insulin resistance and metabolic dysfunction.**

Weight Gain, Obesity, and Insulin Resistance

Excessive weight gain, particularly abdominal obesity, is a key driver on the road to type 2 diabetes. Adipose tissue, especially visceral fat, secretes inflammatory cytokines and adipokines that impair insulin signaling and promote insulin resistance. As weight accumulates, the body's ability to regulate blood sugar becomes compromised, leading to elevated fasting glucose levels and eventually progressing to impaired glucose tolerance and overt diabetes.

Insulin resistance is a hallmark feature of type 2 diabetes and often precedes its diagnosis by years or even decades. Insulin resistance occurs when cells become less responsive to the effects of insulin, leading to impaired glucose uptake and utilization. In response, pancreatic beta cells secrete more insulin to compensate for the reduced sensitivity, resulting in hyperinsulinemia.

Pre-Diabetes and Progression to Diabetes.

Pre-diabetes represents an intermediate stage on the road to type 2 diabetes, characterized by impaired fasting glucose (IFG) and/or impaired glucose tolerance (IGT). Individuals with pre-diabetes have higher-than-normal blood sugar levels but not yet high enough to be diagnosed with diabetes. Without intervention, pre-diabetes often progresses to overt diabetes as beta cell function continues to decline and insulin resistance worsens..It is a **critical window of opportunity** for intervention, as lifestyle modifications and targeted interventions can prevent or delay the progression to diabetes. Lifestyle interventions focused on promoting healthy eating, regular physical activity, weight management, and smoking cessation have been shown to be effective in reducing diabetes risk in individuals with pre-diabetes.

Prediabetes represents an intermediate metabolic state between normal glucose regulation and type 2 diabetes, characterized by higher-than-normal blood sugar levels that are not yet in the diabetic range. Prediabetes is a critical juncture in the progression towards type 2 diabetes and provides an opportunity for early intervention to prevent or delay its onset. Understanding prediabetes and its progression to type 2 diabetes involves exploring the underlying mechanisms, risk factors, diagnostic criteria, management strategies, and implications for public health. They are listed below:

1. Definition and Diagnostic Criteria

Prediabetes encompasses two main categories: **impaired fasting glucose (IFG) and impaired glucose tolerance (IGT).** IFG is defined as fasting blood glucose levels between **100 and 125** mg/dL, while IGT is characterized by elevated blood glucose levels **2 hours after ingesting a standardized glucose solution, typically between 140 and 199 mg/dL on an oral glucose tolerance** test (OGTT). Additionally, hemoglobin **A1c (HbA1c) levels between 5.7% and 6.4%** are also indicative of prediabetes. Diagnosis requires confirmation of elevated blood sugar levels on at least two separate occasions.

2. Underlying Mechanisms

The pathophysiology of prediabetes involves a combination of **insulin resistance and beta-cell dysfunction.** Insulin resistance refers to impaired cellular responsiveness to insulin, resulting in reduced glucose uptake in peripheral tissues such as muscle, liver, and adipose tissue. Beta-cell dysfunction refers to impaired insulin secretion by pancreatic beta cells in response to glucose stimulation. Together, **insulin resistance and beta-cell dysfunction lead to impaired glucose regulation, elevated fasting and postprandial blood glucose levels, and compensatory hyperinsulinemia.** Over time, progressive deterioration in beta-cell function and worsening insulin resistance contribute to the development of overt type 2 diabetes.

3. Risk Factors for Prediabetes:

Several factors increase the risk of developing prediabetes, including obesity, sedentary lifestyle, unhealthy dietary habits, family history of diabetes, ethnicity, age, and history of gestational diabetes. Obesity, particularly central adiposity, is a major driver of insulin resistance and prediabetes, as excess adipose tissue secretes inflammatory cytokines and adipokines that impair insulin signaling and promote metabolic dysfunction. Sedentary behavior further exacerbates insulin resistance, while poor dietary habits characterized by high sugar, refined carbohydrates, and unhealthy fats contribute to dyslipidemia, oxidative stress, and beta-cell dysfunction.

4. Progression to Type 2 Diabetes:

Prediabetes represents a critical stage in the natural history of type 2 diabetes and increases the risk of developing diabetes by **5 to 10 times** compared to individuals with normal glucose tolerance. Without intervention, approximately **15% to 30% of individuals with prediabetes will progress to type 2 diabetes within 5 years, while up to 70% will develop diabetes within their lifetime.** The risk of progression varies based on individual risk factors, with higher risks observed in individuals with **obesity, metabolic syndrome, and severe insulin resistance**. Progressive deterioration in beta-cell function, worsening insulin resistance, and ongoing metabolic dysregulation contribute to the transition from prediabetes to overt diabetes.

5. Management of Prediabetes:

The management of prediabetes focuses on lifestyle modifications aimed at reducing weight, improving dietary habits, increasing physical activity, and promoting smoking cessation. Weight loss of **5% to 10%** of body weight through a combination of caloric restriction and increased physical activity has been shown to significantly reduce the risk of progression to type 2 diabetes and improve metabolic health. Dietary interventions emphasizing a balanced diet rich in fruits, vegetables, whole grains, lean proteins, and healthy fats, while limiting processed foods, sugars, and unhealthy fats, promote weight loss, improve insulin sensitivity, and reduce diabetes risk. Regular physical activity, including aerobic exercise, resistance training, and flexibility exercises, enhances insulin action, promotes weight loss, and improves cardiovascular health. Smoking cessation reduces inflammation, oxidative stress, and cardiovascular risk, further supporting metabolic health. Additionally, pharmacological interventions such as metformin and acarbose may be considered in individuals at high risk of progression to diabetes, particularly those with additional risk factors such as obesity, metabolic syndrome, or history of gestational diabetes.

6. Public Health Implications:

Prediabetes represents a significant public health challenge due to its high prevalence, association with increased diabetes risk, and economic burden on healthcare systems. Early identification and intervention are crucial for preventing or delaying the onset of type 2 diabetes and reducing the burden of diabetes-related complications. Population-based screening programs targeting high-risk individuals, such as those with obesity, metabolic syndrome, or family history of diabetes, can facilitate early detection and intervention. Comprehensive lifestyle interventions delivered through community-based programs, healthcare settings, or digital platforms can empower individuals to make sustainable behavior changes and improve long-term metabolic health. Multisectoral approaches involving healthcare providers, policymakers, employers, schools, and community organizations are needed to create supportive environments that promote healthy lifestyles, prevent obesity, and reduce diabetes risk on a population level.

In conclusion, **prediabetes** represents a critical stage in the progression towards type 2 diabetes and provides a window of opportunity for early intervention to prevent or delay its onset. Understanding the underlying mechanisms, risk factors, diagnostic criteria, management strategies, and public health implications of prediabetes is essential for effective prevention, early detection,

and management of type 2 diabetes. By
implementing evidence-based interventions
targeting lifestyle modifications, population-based
screening, and multisectoral collaboration, we can
mitigate the burden of type 2 diabetes and improve
metabolic health outcomes for individuals and
communities alike.

CHAPTER FOUR

Type 2 diabetes diagnosis, symptoms and complications.

Diagnosis of Type 2 Diabetes

Diagnosing type 2 diabetes involves assessing blood sugar levels through various tests. These tests help healthcare providers determine if a person has diabetes, prediabetes, or normal blood sugar levels. The primary diagnostic tests for type 2 diabetes include:

Fasting Plasma Glucose (FPG) Test: This test measures blood sugar levels after an overnight fast of at least 8 hours. A fasting blood sugar level of 126 milligrams per deciliter (mg/dL) or higher on two separate occasions is diagnostic of diabetes.

Oral Glucose Tolerance Test (OGTT): During this test, blood sugar levels are measured before and 2 hours after drinking a glucose solution. A blood sugar level of 200 mg/dL (11.1 mmol/L) or higher 2 hours after drinking the solution is diagnostic of diabetes.

Hemoglobin A1c (HbA1c) Test: This test measures average blood sugar levels over the past 2-3 months by assessing the percentage of hemoglobin that is glycated (attached to glucose). An A1c level of 6.5% or higher is diagnostic of diabetes.

Random Plasma Glucose Test: This test measures blood sugar levels at any time of day without regard to meals. A random blood sugar level of 200 mg/dL (11.1 mmol/L) or higher, along with symptoms of diabetes, may also be diagnostic of the condition.

Symptoms of Type 2 Diabetes:

Type 2 diabetes often develops gradually, and symptoms may not be noticeable in the early stages. But when the illness worsens, people could have the following signs and symptoms.

- **Increased Thirst (Polydipsia):** Excessive thirst is a common symptom of type 2 diabetes, as high blood sugar levels lead to dehydration.

- **Frequent Urination (Polyuria):** Excess glucose in the bloodstream causes the kidneys to work harder to filter and excrete it, resulting in increased urine production and more frequent trips to the bathroom.

- **Fatigue:** Insulin resistance and impaired glucose metabolism can lead to decreased energy production in cells, resulting in fatigue and feelings of tiredness.

- **Blurry Vision**: High blood sugar levels can cause fluid to be pulled from the lenses of the eyes, resulting in blurry vision or changes in vision.

- **Slow Wound Healing**: Elevated blood sugar levels can impair the body's ability to heal wounds, cuts, and bruises, leading to delayed wound healing.

- **Increased Hunger (Polyphagia)**: Despite eating regularly, individuals with type 2 diabetes may experience persistent hunger due to the body's inability to effectively utilize glucose for energy.

- **Unexplained Weight Loss**: Some individuals with type 2 diabetes may experience unexplained weight loss despite eating more than usual. This can occur due to the body's inability to properly metabolize glucose and utilize it for energy.

- **Numbness or Tingling in Hands or Feet:** Prolonged high blood sugar levels can damage nerves, leading to peripheral neuropathy characterized by numbness, tingling, or burning sensations in the hands or feet.

- **Frequent Infections**: High blood sugar levels weaken the immune system, making individuals with type 2 diabetes more susceptible to infections such as urinary tract infections, skin infections, and yeast infections.

Complications of Type 2 Diabetes:

Untreated or poorly managed type 2 diabetes can lead to a variety of complications that affect nearly every organ system in the body. These complications can be acute or chronic and may include:

- **Cardiovascular Disease**: Individuals with type 2 diabetes are at increased risk of developing cardiovascular disease, including heart attack, stroke, and peripheral artery disease. High blood sugar levels, elevated blood pressure, and abnormal lipid levels contribute to the development of atherosclerosis and increased cardiovascular risk.

- **Nerve Damage (Neuropathy)**: Prolonged high blood sugar levels can damage nerves throughout the body, leading to neuropathy. Peripheral neuropathy affects the nerves in the extremities and can cause symptoms such as numbness, tingling, burning sensations, and pain. Autonomic neuropathy affects the nerves that control involuntary functions such as digestion, heart rate, and blood pressure, leading to symptoms such as gastroparesis, erectile dysfunction, and orthostatic hypotension.

- **Kidney Damage (Nephropathy**): Diabetes is the leading cause of kidney failure, known as diabetic nephropathy. High blood sugar levels and elevated blood pressure can damage the small blood vessels in the kidneys, leading to reduced kidney function and eventually kidney failure.

- **Eye Damage (Retinopathy):** Diabetes can damage the blood vessels in the retina, the light-sensitive tissue at the back of the eye, leading to diabetic retinopathy. This can cause vision problems and eventually blindness if left untreated.

- **Foot Complications:** Diabetes can lead to foot complications such as neuropathy, poor circulation, and impaired wound healing, increasing the risk of foot ulcers and infections. Left untreated, foot ulcers can become infected and may require amputation.

- **Skin Conditions:** Individuals with type 2 diabetes are at increased risk of developing skin conditions such as bacterial and fungal infections, diabetic dermopathy, and necrobiosis lipoidica .

- **Gastroparesis**: Diabetes can affect the nerves that control the muscles of the stomach, leading to delayed gastric emptying and gastroparesis. Symptoms may include nausea, vomiting, bloating, and early satiety.

- **Sexual Dysfunction**: Diabetes can affect sexual function in both men and women. In men, diabetes can cause erectile dysfunction, while in women, it can lead to decreased libido, vaginal dryness, and difficulty achieving orgasm

Conclusion

Type 2 diabetes is a chronic metabolic disorder characterized by elevated blood sugar levels due to insulin resistance and inadequate insulin production. Common symptoms include increased thirst, frequent urination, fatigue, blurry vision, slow wound healing, increased hunger, unexplained weight loss, and numbness or tingling in the hands or feet. Complications of type 2 diabetes can affect nearly every organ system in the body and may include cardiovascular disease, neuropathy, nephropathy, retinopathy, foot complications, skin conditions, gastroparesis, and sexual dysfunction. Early detection and management of type 2 diabetes are crucial for preventing complications and improving long-term health outcomes. Regular monitoring of blood sugar levels, blood pressure, and cholesterol levels, along with lifestyle modifications and appropriate medical management, can help individuals with type 2 diabetes maintain optimal health.

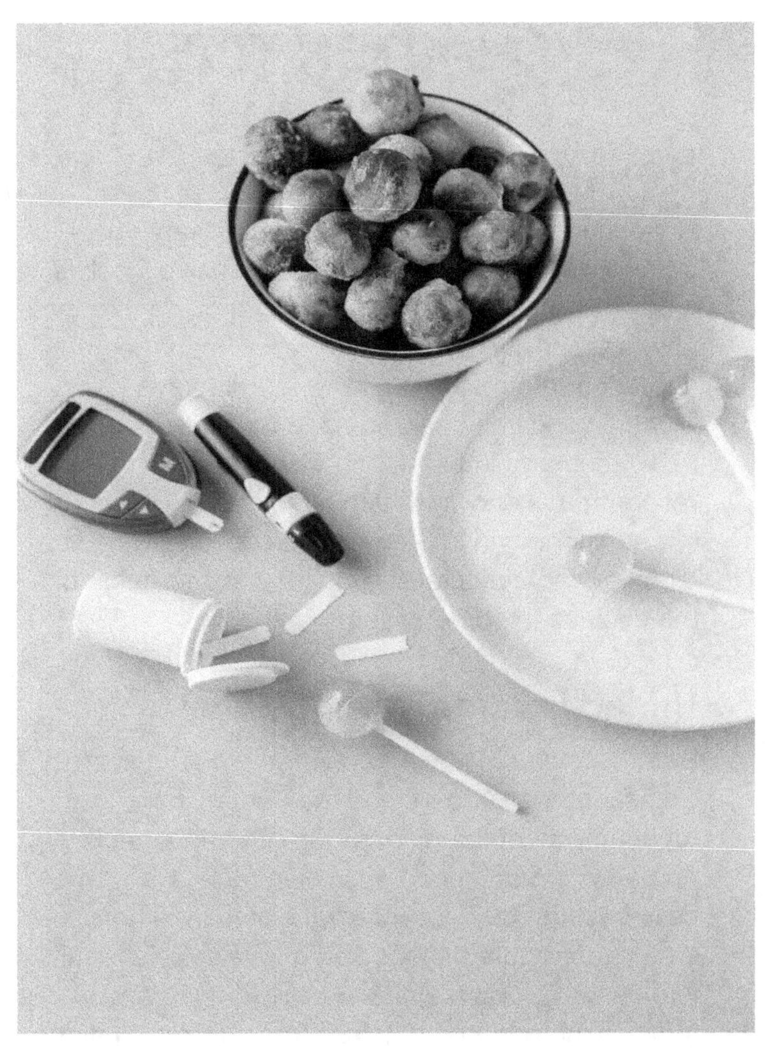

CHAPTER FIVE

REVERSING DIABETES

Reversing type 2 diabetes is an achievable goal for many individuals through comprehensive lifestyle modifications, including dietary changes, increased physical activity, weight loss, stress management, and adequate sleep. While type 2 diabetes is a chronic condition characterized by insulin resistance and impaired glucose metabolism, research has shown that these lifestyle interventions can improve insulin sensitivity, lower blood sugar levels, and even lead to remission of the disease in some cases.

Understanding Type 2 Diabetes:

Before discussing how to reverse type 2 diabetes, it's essential to understand the underlying mechanisms of the disease. Type 2 diabetes is primarily characterized by insulin resistance, where cells become less responsive to insulin, a hormone that helps regulate blood sugar levels. This results in elevated blood sugar levels, leading to symptoms such as increased thirst, frequent urination, fatigue, and blurred vision.

Over time, prolonged exposure to high blood sugar levels can damage organs and tissues throughout the body, leading to complications such as cardiovascular disease, neuropathy, nephropathy, retinopathy, and foot ulcers. However, type 2 diabetes is largely a lifestyle-driven disease, with modifiable risk factors such as obesity, poor diet, sedentary behavior, and stress playing significant roles in its development and progression.

Comprehensive Lifestyle Interventions for Reversing Type 2 Diabetes

DIETARY CHANGES

A balanced, nutrient-dense diet is the cornerstone of diabetes management and reversal. Focus on whole foods such as fruits, vegetables, whole grains, lean proteins, and healthy fats. Emphasize low-glycemic foods that have a minimal impact on blood sugar levels, such as non-starchy vegetables, legumes, nuts, seeds, and whole grains. Limit intake of refined carbohydrates, sugary beverages, processed foods, and high-fat foods, as these can exacerbate insulin resistance and contribute to weight gain. Consider adopting dietary patterns such as the **Mediterranean diet or the DASH (Dietary Approaches to Stop Hypertension) diet,** which have been shown to improve insulin sensitivity and reduce the risk of developing type 2 diabetes.

PHYSICAL ACTIVITY

Regular physical activity is essential for improving insulin sensitivity, lowering blood sugar levels, and promoting weight loss. Aim for at least 150 minutes of moderate-intensity aerobic exercise or 75 minutes of vigorous-intensity exercise per week, along with muscle-strengthening activities on two or more days per week. Choose activities you enjoy, such as walking, cycling, swimming, dancing, or strength training, and incorporate them into your daily routine. Break up long periods of sitting with short bursts of activity, such as standing, stretching, or taking short walks throughout the day.

WEIGHT LOSS

Excess weight, particularly abdominal obesity, is a significant risk factor for type 2 diabetes. Even modest weight loss can improve insulin sensitivity and lead to remission of the disease.

Aim for gradual, sustainable weight loss of 5-10% of your body weight over six to 12 months. This can be achieved through a combination of dietary changes, increased physical activity, and behavior modification. Focus on lifestyle habits rather than short-term fad diets, and aim for long-term behavior change to maintain weight loss and prevent weight regain.

STRESS MANAGEMENT:
Chronic stress can exacerbate insulin resistance and elevate blood sugar levels, so it's essential to incorporate stress-reduction techniques into your daily routine. Practice relaxation techniques such as deep breathing, meditation, yoga, tai chi, or progressive muscle relaxation to reduce stress and promote relaxation. Prioritize self-care activities that bring you joy and relaxation, such as spending time with loved ones, engaging in hobbies, or enjoying nature.

ADEQUATE SLEEP
Poor sleep quality and insufficient sleep duration have been linked to an increased risk of developing type 2 diabetes and worsening blood sugar control in individuals with the disease.
Aim for seven to nine hours of quality sleep per night, and establish a regular sleep schedule by going to bed and waking up at the same time each day. Create a conducive sleep environment by minimizing noise, light, and electronic distractions in the bedroom, and avoid stimulating activities such as screen time before bedtime.

BEHAVIOR MODIFICATION
Changing long-standing habits and behaviors can be challenging, so it's essential to set realistic goals, break tasks into smaller steps, and celebrate small victories along the way. Keep track of your progress by monitoring your food intake, physical

activity, blood sugar levels, weight, and other relevant metrics. This might support your motivation and help you pinpoint areas that need work. Seek support from friends, family members, healthcare professionals, or support groups who can provide encouragement, accountability, and practical advice on how to achieve your goals.

Evidence for Reversing Type 2 Diabetes

Numerous studies have demonstrated the effectiveness of comprehensive lifestyle interventions in reversing type 2 diabetes and achieving glycemic control. One landmark study, the **Diabetes Prevention Program (DPP)**, found that lifestyle changes, including dietary modifications and increased physical activity, reduced the incidence of diabetes by 58% in individuals at high risk for the disease.
Similarly, the **Look AHEAD** (Action for Health in Diabetes) trial showed that intensive lifestyle intervention, consisting of a calorie-restricted diet and increased physical activity, led to greater weight loss, improved glycemic control, and higher rates of diabetes remission compared to standard diabetes support and education programs.

Other studies have highlighted the benefits of specific dietary patterns, such as
low-carbohydrate diets, Mediterranean diets,

and plant-based diets, in improving insulin sensitivity, lowering blood sugar levels, and promoting weight loss in individuals with type 2 diabetes.

MONITORING AND MAINTENANCE:

Monitoring and maintenance are crucial aspects of successfully reversing type 2 diabetes and maintaining long-term glycemic control. After implementing lifestyle modifications and achieving improvements in blood sugar levels, it's essential to continue monitoring your health, staying consistent with healthy habits, and making adjustments as needed to sustain your progress. Here's a detailed guide on monitoring and maintenance in reversing type 2 diabetes:

1. Regular Blood Sugar Monitoring:
Monitor your blood sugar levels regularly using a glucometer or continuous glucose monitoring (CGM) system. This allows you to track your progress, identify patterns, and make adjustments to your lifestyle as needed. Keep a log of your blood sugar readings along with notes on your dietary intake, physical activity, medication use, and any other relevant factors. This information can help you and your healthcare team make informed decisions about your diabetes management.

2. Healthy Eating Habits:
Continue to follow a balanced, nutrient-dense diet
that emphasizes whole foods such as fruits,
vegetables, whole grains, lean proteins, and
healthy fats.
Be mindful of portion sizes, carbohydrate intake,
and the glycemic index of foods to help regulate
blood sugar levels.
Aim for consistency in your eating patterns, sticking
to regular meal times and avoiding skipping meals
or excessive snacking.

3. Regular Physical Activity:
Maintain an active lifestyle by engaging in regular
physical activity, including aerobic exercise,
strength training, and flexibility exercises. Aim for
two or more days of muscle-strengthening
exercises per week in addition to at least 150
minutes of moderate-intensity aerobic exercise or
75 minutes of vigorous-intensity exercise every
week. Find activities that you enjoy and that fit into
your schedule, whether it's walking, cycling,
swimming, dancing, or participating in group fitness
classes.

4. Weight Management
Continue to focus on maintaining a healthy weight
through a combination of dietary modifications,
physical activity, and behavior changes.

Monitor your weight regularly and make adjustments to your lifestyle as needed to prevent weight regain. Be patient and realistic in your weight loss goals, aiming for gradual, sustainable progress over time.

5. Stress Management

Prioritize stress management techniques such as deep breathing, meditation, yoga, tai chi, or progressive muscle relaxation. Practice self-care activities that promote relaxation and well-being, such as spending time with loved ones, engaging in hobbies, or spending time in nature.
Identify sources of stress in your life and develop strategies for coping with them effectively.

6. Adequate Sleep:

Continue to prioritize sleep hygiene and aim for seven to nine hours of quality sleep per night. Stick to a regular sleep schedule by going to bed and waking up at the same time each day, even on weekends. Create a sleep-friendly environment by minimizing noise, light, and electronic distractions in the bedroom.

7. Medication Management:

If you're taking medications for type 2 diabetes, continue to follow your healthcare provider's recommendations and adhere to your prescribed treatment plan. Monitor your blood sugar levels regularly and communicate any changes or concerns to your healthcare team. Be open to adjusting your medication regimen as needed based on changes in your lifestyle, health status, and blood sugar control.

8. Regular Medical Check-ups:
Schedule regular check-ups with your healthcare provider to monitor your overall health and diabetes management. Discuss any concerns or questions you have about your diabetes treatment plan, lifestyle modifications, or potential complications. Stay up to date with recommended screenings, vaccinations, and preventive care measures to optimize your health and well-being.

9. Ongoing Education and Support:
Stay informed about the latest developments in diabetes management, lifestyle interventions, and treatment options. Seek out educational resources, support groups, and online communities where you can connect with others who are on a similar journey. Consider working with a registered dietitian, certified diabetes educator, or other healthcare professionals who can provide guidance, support, and personalized recommendations tailored to your needs.

10. Mindful Eating and Behavior Modification:
Practice mindful eating techniques such as paying
attention to hunger and fullness cues, savoring
each bite, and avoiding distractions while eating.
Be mindful of emotional eating triggers and develop
alternative coping strategies for dealing with stress,
boredom, or other emotions. Use behavior
modification techniques such as goal setting,
self-monitoring, and positive reinforcement to
reinforce healthy habits and overcome challenges.

11. Celebrate Successes and Stay Motivated:
Celebrate your successes, no matter how small,
and acknowledge the progress you've made in
reversing type 2 diabetes. Stay motivated by setting
realistic goals, tracking your progress, and focusing
on the positive changes you've experienced in your
health and well-being. Recognize that setbacks are
a normal part of the journey and use them as
opportunities for learning and growth.
In conclusion, monitoring and maintenance are
essential components of successfully reversing
type 2 diabetes and maintaining long-term glycemic
control. By staying consistent with healthy eating
habits, regular physical activity, stress management
techniques, adequate sleep, medication
management, regular medical check-ups, ongoing
education and support, mindful eating, behavior
modification, and celebrating successes, you can
sustain your progress and enjoy improved health
and well-being for years to come. Remember that

every positive step you take towards better diabetes management brings you closer to achieving your goals and living your best life with type 2 diabetes.

A week food guide on reversing type 2 diabetes

Creating a week-long food guide to reverse type 2 diabetes involves planning balanced meals that emphasize whole foods, limit refined carbohydrates and added sugars, and prioritize nutrient density. Here's a sample food guide for a week to help you manage your blood sugar levels and work towards reversing type 2 diabetes:

Day 1:

Breakfast:
Oatmeal topped with fresh berries, chopped nuts, and a drizzle of honey or a sprinkle of cinnamon.
A side of Greek yogurt or almond milk for added protein.
Lunch:
Grilled chicken salad with mixed greens, cherry tomatoes, cucumber, bell peppers, and avocado.
Dress with olive oil and vinegar or a light vinaigrette dressing.

Snack:
Sliced apple with almond butter or a handful of raw almonds.

Dinner:
Baked salmon filet with steamed broccoli and quinoa. Serve with a squeeze of lemon juice and a sprinkle of fresh herbs.

Day 2:

Breakfast:
Scrambled eggs with spinach, mushrooms, and chopped tomato.
Whole grain toast or a slice of whole wheat bread on the side.

Lunch:
Lentil soup with carrots, celery, onions, and spinach.
Pair with a side of whole grain crackers or a small side salad.

Snack:
Carrot sticks with hummus or a piece of string cheese.

Dinner:
Turkey chili with lean ground turkey, kidney beans, diced tomatoes, onions, and chili spices.
Serve with brown or cauliflower rice for a low-carb option.

Day 3:

Breakfast: Greek yogurt parfait with layers of plain Greek yogurt, sliced bananas, and granola.

Optional: Drizzle with honey or maple syrup for sweetness.

Lunch:

Quinoa salad with mixed greens, chickpeas, roasted vegetables (such as bell peppers, zucchini, and eggplant), and feta cheese.

Toss with olive oil and lemon juice for dressing.

Snack:

Celery sticks with peanut butter or a handful of trail mix (nuts, seeds, and dried fruit).

Dinner:

Stir-fried tofu with mixed vegetables (such as broccoli, bell peppers, snap peas, and carrots) in a light soy sauce or teriyaki sauce.

Serve over brown rice or cauliflower rice.

Day 4:

Breakfast:

Smoothie made with spinach, frozen berries, banana, Greek yogurt, and almond milk.

Optional: add a scoop of protein powder or chia seeds for extra protein and fiber.

Lunch:

Grilled vegetable wrap with hummus, grilled eggplant, zucchini, bell peppers, and onions wrapped in a whole wheat tortilla.

Serve with a side of baby carrots or cucumber slices.

Snack:

Cottage cheese with pineapple chunks or a small handful of walnuts.

Dinner:
Baked chicken breast with roasted sweet potatoes
and steamed green beans.
Season with herbs and spices such as rosemary,
thyme, and garlic.

Day 5:

Breakfast:
Whole grain bread with mashed avocado and sliced
hard-boiled egg sprinkled with salt, pepper, and red
pepper flakes for added flavor.
Lunch:
Spinach salad with grilled shrimp, cherry tomatoes,
cucumbers, and feta cheese.
Dress with a balsamic vinaigrette or lemon tahini
dressing.
Snack:
Edamame (steamed soybeans) or a small handful
of pistachios.
Dinner:
Vegetable stir-fry with tofu or shrimp, bell peppers,
snap peas, broccoli, and carrots in a ginger-garlic
sauce.
Serve over cauliflower rice or brown rice.

Day 6:

Breakfast:
Whole grain cereal with almond milk and sliced
strawberries or blueberries.
Sprinkle with chia seeds or ground flaxseeds for
added fiber.

Lunch:
Turkey and avocado wrap with whole wheat tortilla, sliced turkey breast, avocado, lettuce, tomato, and mustard. Serve with a side of baby carrots or sliced bell peppers.
Snack:
Greek yogurt with a drizzle of honey or a sprinkle of granola.
Dinner:
Baked cod with roasted Brussels sprouts and quinoa pilaf.
Season cod with lemon, garlic, and herbs such as dill or parsley.

Day 7:

Breakfast:
Veggie omelet with spinach, mushrooms, onions, and bell peppers.
Serve with a side of whole grain toast or fruit salad.
Lunch:
Black bean and vegetable soup with diced tomatoes, onions, carrots, celery, and bell peppers. Garnish with cilantro and a dollop of Greek yogurt or sour cream.
Snack:
Sliced cucumber with tzatziki sauce or a small handful of mixed berries.
Dinner:
Grilled steak or portobello mushrooms with roasted asparagus and mashed cauliflower.

Season steak with salt, pepper, and your favorite herbs, and mash cauliflower with garlic and olive oil.

Tips for Success:

- Maintain hydration by drinking plenty of water throughout the day.
- Choose snacks that are high in fiber, protein, and healthy fats to keep you feeling full and satisfied.
- Experiment with herbs, spices, and different cooking techniques to add flavor to your meals without relying on added sugars or salt.
- Practice portion control and mindful eating by paying attention to hunger and fullness cues.
- Be consistent with your mealtimes and eating patterns to help regulate blood sugar levels and optimize digestion.

CHAPTER SIX

THE DECISIVE MOMENT

Reversing type 2 diabetes is a significant achievement that can lead to improved health, well-being, and quality of life. After adhering to the tips and guidelines for managing and reversing type 2 diabetes, individuals often experience a turning point where they notice positive changes in their health, energy levels, and overall outlook on life. Here are some common decisive moments that individuals may experience on their journey to reversing type 2 diabetes:

1. IMPROVED BLOOD SUGAR CONTROL

One of the most significant moments for individuals with type 2 diabetes is seeing improvements in their blood sugar levels. With consistent lifestyle modifications, including dietary changes, regular physical activity, and weight loss, many people experience more stable and normalized blood sugar readings.

They may notice fewer spikes and dips in blood sugar levels throughout the day, leading to fewer symptoms of hyperglycemia (high blood sugar) and hypoglycemia (low blood sugar).

2. REDUCTION IN MEDICATION USE

As blood sugar levels improve, some individuals may experience a reduction in the need for diabetes medications or insulin. Their healthcare provider may adjust their medication regimen, lower dosages, or even discontinue certain medications altogether.

This reduction in medication use can be empowering and signify a significant milestone in managing their diabetes effectively through lifestyle changes.

3. INCREASED ENERGY AND VITALITY

Many individuals report feeling more energetic, alert, and vibrant after implementing healthy lifestyle habits to manage their diabetes. They may notice improvements in their overall energy levels, mental clarity, and ability to engage in daily activities without fatigue or lethargy.

With better blood sugar control and improved insulin sensitivity, cells throughout the body can better utilize glucose for energy, leading to increased vitality and well-being.

4. Weight Loss and Body Composition Changes

Weight loss is often a key component of reversing type 2 diabetes, and many individuals experience significant changes in their body composition as they adopt healthier habits. They may notice a decrease in body fat, particularly abdominal fat, and an increase in lean muscle mass.

Achieving and maintaining a healthy weight can improve insulin sensitivity, reduce inflammation, and lower the risk of obesity-related health conditions, such as heart disease and stroke.

5. Better Management of Other Health Conditions

Type 2 diabetes is often accompanied by other health conditions, such as high blood pressure, high cholesterol, and fatty liver disease. As individuals make lifestyle changes to manage their diabetes, they may also see improvements in these coexisting conditions.
Better management of these comorbidities can lead to a lower risk of complications and an overall improvement in health and longevity.

6. SENSE OF EMPOWERMENT AND CONTROL

Reversing type 2 diabetes requires dedication, commitment, and perseverance, and achieving this goal can instill a profound sense of empowerment and control over one's health.
Individuals may feel empowered to take charge of their health and make informed decisions about their lifestyle, diet, exercise, and overall well-being.

7. ENHANCED QUALITY OF LIFE:

Ultimately, the turning point after reversing type 2 diabetes is experiencing an enhanced quality of life. Individuals may enjoy improved physical health, mental well-being, and emotional resilience, allowing them to fully engage in and enjoy life's activities.

They may feel more confident, optimistic, and hopeful about the future, knowing that they have the power to manage their diabetes and live a fulfilling life.

8. INSPIRATION FOR OTHERS:
Lastly, individuals who successfully reverse type 2 diabetes may become sources of inspiration and encouragement for others facing similar challenges. By sharing their journey, insights, and successes, they can motivate and support others on their path to better health and wellness.

In conclusion, the turning point after adhering to tips for reversing type 2 diabetes is experiencing positive changes in blood sugar control, medication use, energy levels, body composition, overall health, empowerment, and quality of life. It's a transformative journey that requires commitment, but the rewards are immense and can inspire others to embark on their own paths to better health.

CHAPTER SEVEN

Summary

Reversing type 2 diabetes involves adopting lifestyle changes aimed at managing blood sugar levels effectively. This condition, characterized by insulin resistance and impaired glucose regulation, can be mitigated through a combination of dietary adjustments, increased physical activity, weight management, and sometimes medication.

Dietary changes play a central role in reversing type 2 diabetes. This often involves reducing the intake of refined sugars and carbohydrates while focusing on whole, nutrient-dense foods such as fruits, vegetables, lean proteins, and healthy fats. The emphasis is on controlling portion sizes and eating meals with a balanced macronutrient composition to prevent spikes in blood sugar levels.

Regular physical activity is another key component in diabetes management and reversal. Exercise improves insulin sensitivity, allowing cells to more efficiently use glucose for energy. Both aerobic exercises, like walking, swimming, and cycling, and resistance training can be beneficial. Aim for at least 150 minutes of moderate-intensity activity every week, spaced out over many days.

Weight management is closely linked to diabetes reversal, as excess body fat contributes to insulin resistance. Achieving and maintaining a healthy weight through a combination of diet and exercise can significantly improve blood sugar control and may even lead to remission of the condition in some cases.

In addition to lifestyle modifications, medication may be prescribed to help lower blood sugar levels and improve insulin sensitivity. This could include oral medications such as metformin or insulin injections in more severe cases. However, medication should be seen as a complement to, rather than a substitute for, lifestyle changes.

Regular monitoring of blood sugar levels is essential to track progress and make necessary adjustments to the treatment plan. This may involve self-monitoring at home using a glucometer or periodic tests conducted by healthcare professionals.

Overall, reversing type 2 diabetes requires a holistic approach that addresses multiple aspects of health and wellness. By adopting healthy eating habits, engaging in regular physical activity, managing weight, and working closely with healthcare providers, individuals with type 2 diabetes can improve their quality of life and potentially achieve remission of the condition. It's important to recognize that while diabetes reversal is achievable for some, it may not be possible for everyone, and ongoing management is essential for long-term health.

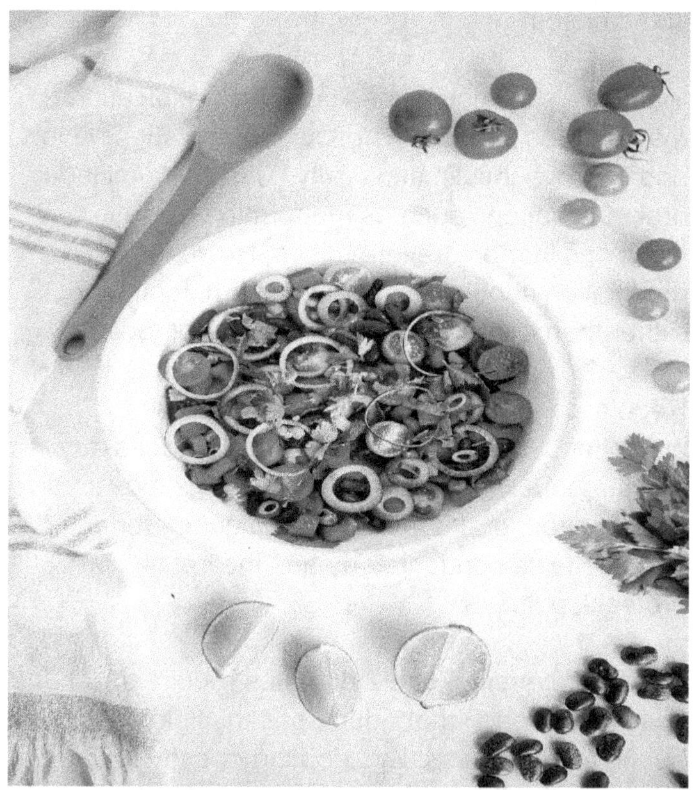

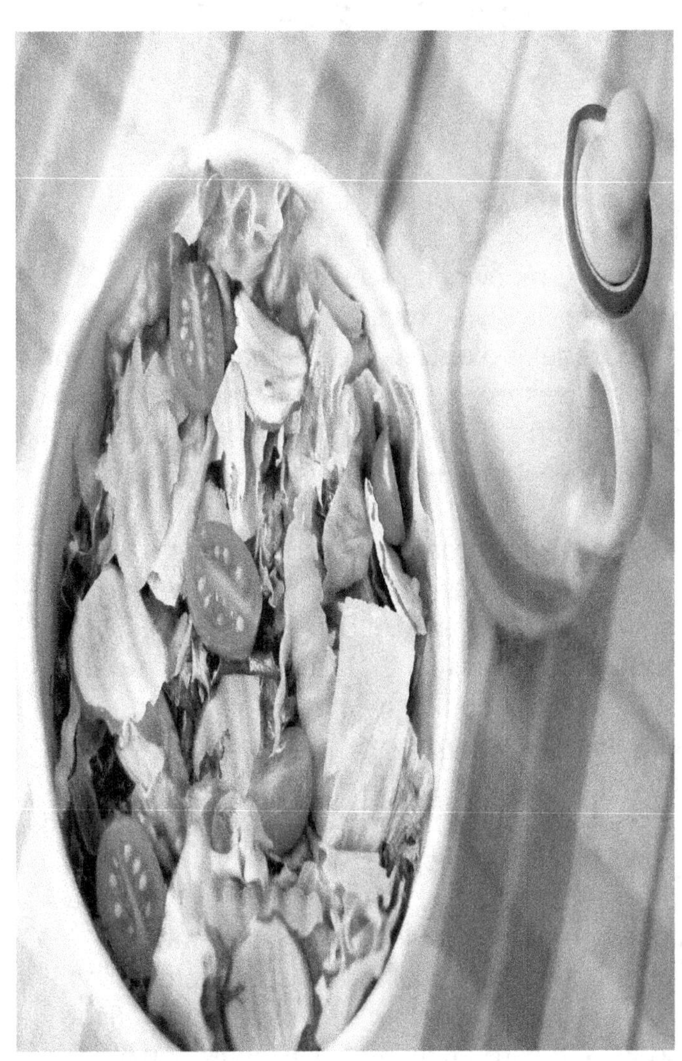

CHAPTER EIGHT

CONCLUSION

In conclusion, the journey to reversing type 2 diabetes is indeed challenging, but it is also incredibly empowering and rewarding. By embracing lifestyle changes that prioritize healthy eating, regular exercise, weight management, and, when necessary, medication, individuals with type 2 diabetes can take control of their health and potentially achieve remission of the condition.

The path to diabetes reversal begins with a shift in mindset – from viewing diabetes as an insurmountable obstacle to seeing it as a manageable condition that can be overcome with determination and commitment. This shift is supported by a wealth of scientific evidence demonstrating the effectiveness of lifestyle interventions in improving blood sugar control and promoting overall well-being.

At the heart of diabetes reversal is dietary modification. By choosing whole, nutrient-dense foods and minimizing the consumption of refined sugars and carbohydrates, individuals can stabilize blood sugar levels and reduce insulin resistance. This approach not only improves metabolic health but also nourishes the body with essential vitamins, minerals, and antioxidants, supporting overall vitality.

Physical activity is another cornerstone of diabetes reversal. Regular exercise not only helps to lower blood sugar levels but also enhances insulin sensitivity, allowing cells to more effectively utilize glucose for energy. Whether it's walking, swimming, cycling, or strength training, finding enjoyable ways to stay active is key to long-term success.

Weight management plays a pivotal role in diabetes reversal, as excess body fat is closely linked to insulin resistance. Through a combination of healthy eating and regular exercise, individuals can achieve and maintain a healthy weight, reducing the burden on their bodies and improving metabolic function.

While lifestyle changes are fundamental to diabetes reversal, medication may also be necessary to achieve optimal blood sugar control. Medications such as metformin or insulin therapy may be prescribed to complement lifestyle interventions and help individuals reach their treatment goals. It's important to work closely with healthcare providers to find the right combination of treatments tailored to individual needs.

Throughout the journey to diabetes reversal, regular monitoring of blood sugar levels is essential. This allows individuals to track their progress, identify areas for improvement, and make necessary adjustments to their treatment plan. With the support of healthcare professionals, individuals can feel confident in their ability to manage their condition and achieve their health goals.

Ultimately, the journey to reversing type 2 diabetes is about reclaiming control over one's health and well-being. It's about making empowered choices that prioritize self-care and vitality. While the road may have its challenges, the destination – a life free from the constraints of diabetes – is well worth the effort.

In the end, achieving diabetes reversal is not just about reaching a specific blood sugar target; it's about reclaiming a sense of freedom, vitality, and peace of mind. It's about embracing a new way of living that nourishes the body, nurtures the spirit, and celebrates the incredible resilience of the human spirit. With determination, support, and a commitment to self-care, individuals with type 2 diabetes can rewrite their health narrative and embrace a brighter, healthier future.

BONUS: A 14- DAY MEAL PLAN REMARK

DAY	MEAL	REMARK